COMPLETE RENAL DIET

COOKBOOK

Nourish Your Kidneys with Delectable Low-Sodium, Low-Potassium, and Low-Phosphorus Recipes

T. John

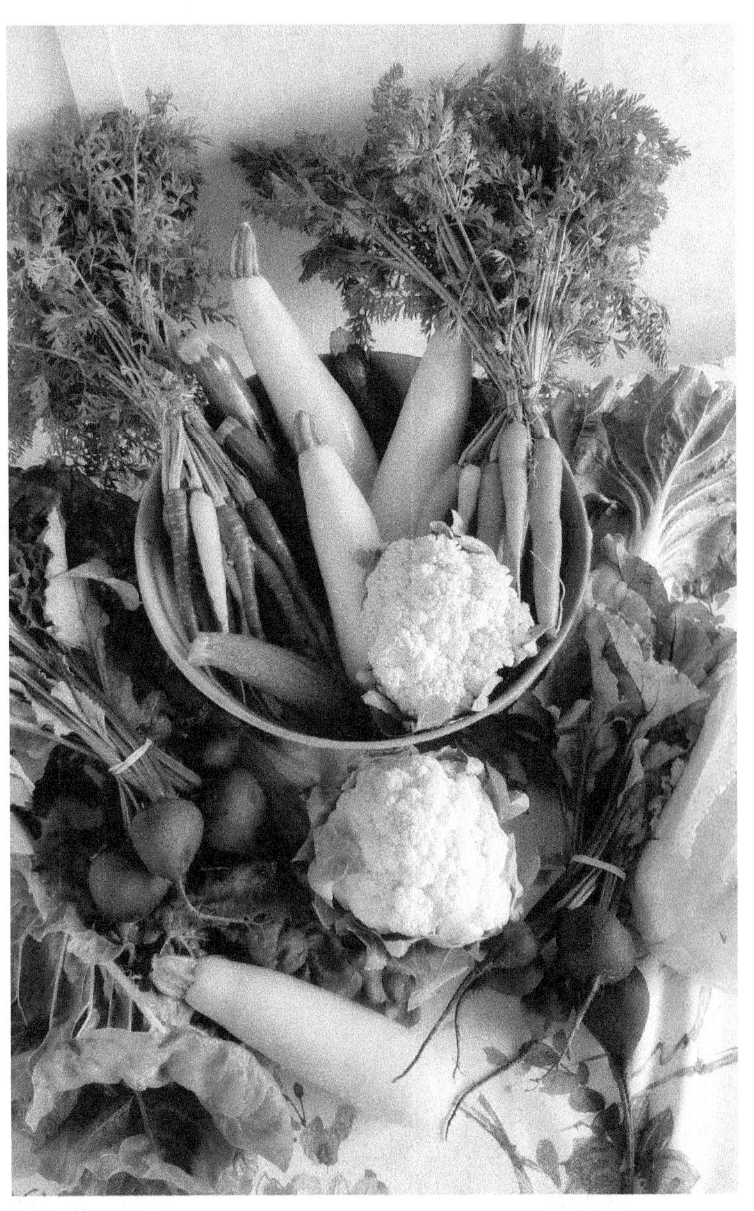

TABLE OF CONTENTS

Chapter 3: Lunch Recipes 39

Chapter 4: Dinner Recipes 56

Chapter 5: Snacks and Appetizers 76

INTRODUCTION

For individuals with chronic kidney disease (CKD), managing their diet is crucial. A renal diet, also known as a kidney-friendly diet, is specifically designed to support kidney function and slow disease progression.

What is a renal diet?

A renal diet is a personalized dietary plan that is tailored to your specific needs and stage of CKD. It typically focuses on:

- Limiting protein: Protein breakdown produces waste products that the kidneys need to filter. In CKD, limiting protein can help reduce the workload on the kidneys and protect them from further damage.
- Controlling phosphorus: Phosphorus is a mineral found in many foods that can build up in the blood and contribute to bone disease in individuals with CKD. A renal diet limits phosphorus intake to help manage blood levels.

- Restricting sodium: Sodium can contribute to high blood pressure, a common complication of CKD. A renal diet typically limits sodium intake to help control blood pressure and reduce strain on the kidneys.

- Balancing potassium: Potassium is another mineral that can build up in the blood in individuals with CKD. A renal diet may limit or encourage potassium intake depending on individual needs.

Why is a renal diet important?

Following a renal diet offers numerous benefits for individuals with CKD, including:

- Slower disease progression: By limiting waste products and toxins in the blood, a renal diet can help slow the progression of CKD and delay the need for dialysis or a kidney transplant.

- Improved symptom management: A renal diet can help manage symptoms of CKD, such as fatigue,nausea, and weakness.

- Reduced risk of complications: A renal diet can help reduce the risk of CKD-related complications, such as heart disease, bone disease, and anemia.
- Improved quality of life: By managing their diet and feeling better, individuals with CKD can experience a better quality of life.

Tips for successful implementation of a renal diet:

- Set realistic goals: Start with small changes and gradually make them a part of your lifestyle.
- Plan your meals and snacks:Planning meals and snacks ahead of time can help you stay on track and avoid unhealthy choices.
- Cook more meals at home: This gives you more control over the ingredients and portion sizes in your food.
- Read food labels carefully: Pay attention to the serving size and the amount of protein, phosphorus,sodium, and potassium in each serving.

- Find healthy alternatives: There are many delicious and healthy alternatives to your favorite foods that are still kidney-friendly.

- Get support from friends and family: Let your loved ones know about your new diet and ask them for their support.

- Join a support group: Connecting with other individuals with CKD can provide valuable support and encouragement.

By understanding the importance of a renal diet and following these tips for successful implementation, you can take control of your CKD and improve your quality of life.

Chapter 1: 30-Day Meal Plan

Week 1:

Day 1:

- Breakfast: Healthy Quinoa Breakfast Bowl
- Lunch: Lentil and Vegetable Soup
- Dinner: Baked Cod with Lemon and Herbs
- Snack: Hummus with Veggie Sticks
- Dessert: Berry and Yogurt Parfait

Day 2:

- Breakfast: Spinach and Feta Omelette
- Lunch: Grilled Chicken Salad
- Dinner: Eggplant Parmesan
- Snack: Guacamole with Whole Grain Chips
- Dessert: Mango Sorbet

Day 3:

- Breakfast: Berry Parfait
- Lunch: Quinoa and Black Bean Bowl
- Dinner: Chicken and Vegetable Skewers

- Snack: Greek Yogurt and Cucumber Dip
- Dessert: Dark Chocolate Avocado Mousse

Day 4:

- Breakfast: Avocado Toast with Poached Egg
- Lunch: Salmon and Asparagus Parcels
- Dinner: Quinoa-Stuffed Bell Peppers
- Snack: Mixed Nuts and Seeds
- Dessert: Baked Apple with Cinnamon

Day 5:

- Breakfast: Banana Walnut Pancakes
- Lunch: Turkey and Vegetable Stir-Fry
- Dinner: Teriyaki Salmon with Vegetables
- Snack: Stuffed Grape Leaves
- Dessert: Chia Seed Pudding with Berries

Day 6:

- Breakfast: Veggie Frittata
- Lunch: Caprese Salad with Balsamic Glaze
- Dinner: Turkey and Quinoa Meatballs
- Snack: Baked Sweet Potato Fries

- Dessert: Almond and Coconut Energy Bites

Day 7:

- Breakfast: Overnight Chia Pudding
- Lunch: Chickpea and Spinach Curry
- Dinner: Vegetable and Lentil Curry
- Snack: Edamame with Sea Salt
- Dessert: Greek Yogurt and Honey Tart

Week 2:

Day 8:

- Breakfast: Sweet Potato Hash
- Lunch: Shrimp and Quinoa Salad
- Dinner: Grilled Swordfish with Mango Salsa
- Snack: Caprese Skewers
- Dessert: Watermelon Granita

Day 9:

- Breakfast: Greek Yogurt with Berries
- Lunch: Sweet Potato and Kale Salad
- Dinner: Spinach and Ricotta Stuffed Chicken Breast
- Snack: Roasted Chickpeas

- Dessert: Poached Pears in Red Wine

Day 10:

- Breakfast: Egg and Vegetable Muffins
- Lunch: Ratatouille with Brown Rice
- Dinner: Portobello Mushroom Steaks
- Snack: Avocado Bruschetta
- Dessert: Pistachio and Cranberry Bark

Day 11:

- Breakfast: Oatmeal with Mixed Berries
- Lunch: Tofu and Broccoli Stir-Fry
- Dinner: Pesto Zoodles with Cherry Tomatoes
- Snack: Spicy Tuna Lettuce Wraps
- Dessert: Pumpkin Pie Smoothie Bowl

Day 12:

- Breakfast: Cottage Cheese and Pineapple Bowl
- Lunch: Caesar Salad with Grilled Chicken
- Dinner: Black Bean and Vegetable Stir-Fry
- Snack: Cottage Cheese and Tomato Slices
- Dessert: Blueberry Oat Bars

Day 13:

- Breakfast: Whole Grain Waffles
- Lunch: Mediterranean Chickpea Wrap
- Dinner: Baked Chicken with Rosemary
- Snack: Sliced Apple with Almond Butter
- Dessert: Peach and Berry Cobbler

Day 14:

- Breakfast: Mediterranean Breakfast Wrap
- Lunch: Zucchini Noodles with Pesto
- Dinner: Cauliflower and Chickpea Curry
- Snack: Veggie Spring Rolls
- Dessert: Lemon Poppy Seed Muffins

Week 3:

Day 15:

- Breakfast: Healthy Quinoa Breakfast Bowl
- Lunch: Lentil and Vegetable Soup
- Dinner: Baked Cod with Lemon and Herbs
- Snack: Hummus with Veggie Sticks
- Dessert: Berry and Yogurt Parfait

Day 16:

- Breakfast: Spinach and Feta Omelette
- Lunch: Grilled Chicken Salad
- Dinner: Eggplant Parmesan
- Snack: Guacamole with Whole Grain Chips
- Dessert: Mango Sorbet

Day 17:

- Breakfast: Berry Parfait
- Lunch: Quinoa and Black Bean Bowl
- Dinner: Chicken and Vegetable Skewers
- Snack: Greek Yogurt and Cucumber Dip
- Dessert: Dark Chocolate Avocado Mousse

Day 18:

- Breakfast: Avocado Toast with Poached Egg
- Lunch: Salmon and Asparagus Parcels
- Dinner: Quinoa-Stuffed Bell Peppers
- Snack: Mixed Nuts and Seeds
- Dessert: Baked Apple with Cinnamon

Day 19:

- Breakfast: Banana Walnut Pancakes
- Lunch: Turkey and Vegetable Stir-Fry
- Dinner: Teriyaki Salmon with Vegetables
- Snack: Stuffed Grape Leaves
- Dessert: Chia Seed Pudding with Berries

Day 20:

- Breakfast: Veggie Frittata
- Lunch: Caprese Salad with Balsamic Glaze
- Dinner: Turkey and Quinoa Meatballs
- Snack: Baked Sweet Potato Fries
- Dessert: Almond and Coconut Energy Bites

Day 21:

- Breakfast: Overnight Chia Pudding
- Lunch: Chickpea and Spinach Curry
- Dinner: Vegetable and Lentil Curry
- Snack: Edamame with Sea Salt
- Dessert: Greek Yogurt and Honey Tart

Week 4:

Day 22:

- Breakfast: Sweet Potato Hash
- Lunch: Shrimp and Quinoa Salad
- Dinner: Grilled Swordfish with Mango Salsa
- Snack: Caprese Skewers
- Dessert: Watermelon Granita

Day 23:

- Breakfast: Greek Yogurt with Berries
- Lunch: Sweet Potato and Kale Salad
- Dinner: Spinach and Ricotta Stuffed Chicken Breast
- Snack: Roasted Chickpeas
- Dessert: Poached Pears in Red Wine

Day 24:

- Breakfast: Egg and Vegetable Muffins
- Lunch: Ratatouille with Brown Rice
- Dinner: Portobello Mushroom Steaks
- Snack: Avocado Bruschetta
- Dessert: Pistachio and Cranberry Bark

Day 25:

- Breakfast: Oatmeal with Mixed Berries
- Lunch: Tofu and Broccoli Stir-Fry
- Dinner: Pesto Zoodles with Cherry Tomatoes
- Snack: Spicy Tuna Lettuce Wraps
- Dessert: Pumpkin Pie Smoothie Bowl

Day 26:

- Breakfast: Cottage Cheese and Pineapple Bowl
- Lunch: Caesar Salad with Grilled Chicken
- Dinner: Black Bean and Vegetable Stir-Fry
- Snack: Cottage Cheese and Tomato Slices
- Dessert: Blueberry Oat Bars

Day 27:

- Breakfast: Whole Grain Waffles
- Lunch: Mediterranean Chickpea Wrap
- Dinner: Baked Chicken with Rosemary
- Snack: Sliced Apple with Almond Butter
- Dessert: Peach and Berry Cobbler

Day 28:

- Breakfast: Mediterranean Breakfast Wrap
- Lunch: Zucchini Noodles with Pesto
- Dinner: Cauliflower and Chickpea Curry
- Snack: Veggie Spring Rolls
- Dessert: Lemon Poppy Seed Muffins

Day 29:

- Breakfast: Healthy Quinoa Breakfast Bowl
- Lunch: Lentil and Vegetable Soup
- Dinner: Baked Cod with Lemon and Herbs
- Snack: Hummus with Veggie Sticks
- Dessert: Berry and Yogurt Parfait

Day 30:

- Breakfast: Spinach and Feta Omelette
- Lunch: Grilled Chicken Salad
- Dinner: Eggplant Parmesan
- Snack: Guacamole with Whole Grain Chips
- Dessert: Mango Sorbet

Feel free to adjust the plan based on your preferences and dietary needs. Enjoy your 30-day renal diet meal plan!

Chapter 2: Breakfast Recipes

Start your day right with a collection of nourishing breakfast recipes that not only tantalize your taste buds but also prioritize your health. These breakfast ideas are crafted to provide a perfect balance of flavors and nutrients, ensuring a wholesome start to your morning routine. From hearty quinoa bowls to delightful fruit parfaits, each recipe is designed with care to make your breakfast a delightful experience.

Healthy Quinoa Breakfast Bowl

Ingredients:

- 1 cup cooked quinoa
- 1/2 cup Greek yogurt
- 1/4 cup fresh berries (strawberries, blueberries, or raspberries)
- 1 tablespoon honey
- 1 tablespoon chopped nuts (almonds, walnuts, or pistachios)

Instructions:

1. In a bowl, layer cooked quinoa.

2. Top with Greek yogurt and fresh berries.

3. Drizzle with honey and sprinkle chopped nuts.

4. Enjoy this protein-packed breakfast bowl!

Nutrition Information:

Calories: 350 | Protein: 15g | Carbohydrates: 55g | Fat: 10g

Portion Size: 1 serving

Spinach and Feta Omelette

Ingredients:

- 2 eggs

- Handful of fresh spinach

- 1/4 cup crumbled feta cheese

- Salt and pepper to taste

- 1 teaspoon olive oil

Instructions:

1. Whisk eggs and season with salt and pepper.

2. Heat olive oil in a pan, add spinach until wilted.

3. Pour eggs over spinach, sprinkle feta, and cook until set.

4. Fold and serve this nutritious omelette.

Nutrition Information:

Calories: 280 | Protein: 18g | Carbohydrates: 4g | Fat: 21g

Portion Size: 1 serving

Berry Parfait

Ingredients:

- 1/2 cup Greek yogurt
- 1/2 cup mixed berries (strawberries, blueberries, and raspberries)
- 2 tablespoons granola
- 1 teaspoon honey

Instructions:

1. Layer Greek yogurt, mixed berries, and granola in a glass.

2. Repeat the layers and drizzle with honey.

3. Revel in the delightful flavors of this berry parfait.

Nutrition Information:

Calories: 220 | Protein: 10g | Carbohydrates: 35g | Fat: 5g

Portion Size: 1 serving

Avocado Toast with Poached Egg

Ingredients:

- 1 slice whole-grain bread
- 1/2 ripe avocado
- 1 poached egg
- Salt and pepper to taste
- Red pepper flakes (optional)

Instructions:

1. Toast the bread and spread avocado on top.
2. Place a poached egg on the avocado.
3. Season with salt, pepper, and red pepper flakes if desired.
4. Dive into the creamy goodness of this nutritious toast.

Nutrition Information:

Calories: 280 | Protein: 12g | Carbohydrates: 20g | Fat: 18g

Portion Size: 1 serving

Banana Walnut Pancakes

Ingredients:

- 1 cup whole wheat flour
- 1 ripe banana, mashed
- 1/2 cup chopped walnuts
- 1 teaspoon baking powder
- 1 cup milk (or plant-based milk)
- 1 egg
- 1 tablespoon maple syrup

Instructions:

1. In a bowl, mix flour, banana, walnuts, and baking powder.
2. Add milk, egg, and maple syrup, stirring until smooth.
3. Cook spoonfuls of batter on a griddle until golden.
4. Serve these fluffy pancakes with a drizzle of maple syrup.

Nutrition Information:

Calories: 320 | Protein: 10g | Carbohydrates: 45g | Fat: 12g

Portion Size: 2-3 pancakes

Veggie Frittata

Ingredients:

- 4 eggs
- 1/2 cup diced bell peppers
- 1/2 cup cherry tomatoes, halved
- 1/4 cup chopped spinach
- 1/4 cup feta cheese
- Salt and pepper to taste
- 1 teaspoon olive oil

Instructions:

1. Whisk eggs and season with salt and pepper.
2. Sauté veggies in olive oil until tender.
3. Pour eggs over veggies, sprinkle with feta, and cook until set.
4. Slice and savor this colorful veggie frittata.

Nutrition Information:

Calories: 250 | Protein: 15g | Carbohydrates: 7g | Fat: 18g

Portion Size: 1 serving

Overnight Chia Pudding

Ingredients:

- 2 tablespoons chia seeds
- 1/2 cup almond milk
- 1/2 teaspoon vanilla extract
- 1 tablespoon maple syrup
- Fresh berries for topping

Instructions:

1. Mix chia seeds, almond milk, vanilla, and maple syrup in a jar.
2. Refrigerate overnight or at least 4 hours until thickened.
3. Top with fresh berries before serving.
4. Enjoy this effortless and nutritious chia pudding.

Nutrition Information:

Calories: 180 | Protein: 5g | Carbohydrates: 20g | Fat: 9g

Portion Size: 1 serving

Blueberry Almond Smoothie Bowl

Ingredients:

- 1 cup frozen blueberries
- 1/2 banana
- 1/2 cup almond milk
- 1 tablespoon almond butter
- Toppings: sliced almonds, fresh blueberries

Instructions:

1. Blend blueberries, banana, almond milk, and almond butter until smooth.
2. Pour into a bowl and top with sliced almonds and fresh blueberries.
3. Indulge in the vibrant flavors of this nourishing smoothie bowl.

Nutrition Information:

Calories: 250 | Protein: 8g | Carbohydrates: 35g | Fat: 10g

Portion Size: 1 serving

Sweet Potato Hash

Ingredients:

- 1 medium sweet potato, diced
- 1/2 onion, chopped
- 1 bell pepper, diced
- 1 tablespoon olive oil
- 1 teaspoon paprika
- Salt and pepper to taste

Instructions:

1. In a skillet, sauté sweet potato, onion, and bell pepper in olive oil.
2. Season with paprika, salt, and pepper.
3. Cook until sweet potatoes are tender and slightly crispy.
4. Serve this savory sweet potato hash for a hearty breakfast.

Nutrition Information:

Calories: 220 | Protein: 3g | Carbohydrates: 35g | Fat: 8g

Portion Size: 1 serving

Greek Yogurt with Berries

Ingredients:

- 1 cup Greek yogurt
- Mixed berries (strawberries, blueberries, raspberries)
- 1 tablespoon honey
- Granola for crunch

Instructions:

1. Spoon Greek yogurt into a bowl.
2. Top with mixed berries, drizzle with honey, and add granola.
3. Enjoy the creamy and fruity goodness of this yogurt bowl.

Nutrition Information:

Calories: 280 | Protein: 15g | Carbohydrates: 30g | Fat: 12g

Portion Size: 1 serving

Egg and Vegetable Muffins

Ingredients:

- 4 eggs

- 1/2 cup diced bell peppers
- 1/2 cup diced zucchini
- 1/4 cup shredded cheddar cheese
- Salt and pepper to taste
- Cooking spray

Instructions:

1. Preheat oven to 350°F (175°C) and grease a muffin tin with cooking spray.
2. In a bowl, whisk eggs and season with salt and pepper.
3. Stir in bell peppers, zucchini, and cheddar cheese.
4. Pour mixture into muffin cups and bake for 20-25 minutes.
5. Enjoy these flavorful and portable egg and vegetable muffins.

Nutrition Information:

Calories: 180 | Protein: 12g | Carbohydrates: 5g | Fat: 12g

Portion Size: 2 muffins

Oatmeal with Mixed Berries

Ingredients:

- 1/2 cup rolled oats
- 1 cup milk (or plant-based milk)
- Mixed berries (strawberries, blueberries, raspberries)
- 1 tablespoon honey
- Chopped nuts for crunch

Instructions:

1. Cook oats in milk according to package instructions.
2. Top with mixed berries, drizzle with honey, and add chopped nuts.
3. Savor the comforting warmth and flavors of this oatmeal bowl.

Nutrition Information:

Calories: 220 | Protein: 8g | Carbohydrates: 35g | Fat: 6g

Portion Size: 1 serving

Cottage Cheese and Pineapple Bowl

Ingredients:

- 1 cup low-fat cottage cheese
- 1/2 cup diced pineapple
- 1 tablespoon chia seeds
- 1 tablespoon shredded coconut

Instructions:

1. In a bowl, combine cottage cheese and diced pineapple.
2. Sprinkle chia seeds and shredded coconut on top.
3. Mix well and relish the tropical goodness of this cottage cheese bowl.

Nutrition Information:

Calories: 220 | Protein: 20g | Carbohydrates: 15g | Fat: 8g

Portion Size: 1 serving

Whole Grain Waffles

Ingredients:

- 1 cup whole wheat flour

- 1 tablespoon baking powder
- 1 tablespoon honey
- 1 cup milk (or plant-based milk)
- 1 egg
- Fresh fruit for topping

Instructions:

1. Mix whole wheat flour, baking powder, honey, milk, and egg in a bowl.
2. Pour batter onto a preheated waffle iron and cook until golden.
3. Top with fresh fruit for a wholesome and delicious breakfast.

Nutrition Information:

Calories: 280 | Protein: 10g | Carbohydrates: 45g | Fat: 8g

Portion Size: 2 waffles

Mediterranean Breakfast Wrap

Ingredients:

- 1 whole-grain tortilla
- 2 eggs, scrambled

- 1/4 cup diced tomatoes
- 1/4 cup diced cucumbers
- 2 tablespoons feta cheese, crumbled
- Fresh parsley for garnish
- Salt and pepper to taste

Instructions:

1. Heat the tortilla in a pan or microwave until warm.
2. Scramble the eggs and season with salt and pepper.
3. Place the scrambled eggs on the tortilla.
4. Top with diced tomatoes, cucumbers, and crumbled feta.
5. Garnish with fresh parsley, fold, and enjoy this Mediterranean-inspired breakfast wrap.

Nutrition Information:

Calories: 320 | Protein: 18g | Carbohydrates: 25g | Fat: 15g

Portion Size: 1 serving

Chapter 3: Lunch Recipes

Embark on a delightful culinary journey with our collection of vibrant and nourishing lunch recipes. From hearty soups to crisp salads and flavorful stir-fries, this chapter is designed to tantalize your taste buds while keeping your nutritional needs in mind. Each recipe is crafted with a balance of wholesome ingredients, offering a variety of flavors and textures to make your midday meals a delightful experience.

Lentil and Vegetable Soup

Ingredients:

- 1 cup green lentils
- 2 carrots, diced
- 1 onion, chopped
- 3 cloves garlic, minced
- 1 zucchini, sliced
- 4 cups vegetable broth
- 1 teaspoon cumin
- Salt and pepper to taste

Instructions:

1. In a large pot, sauté onions and garlic until fragrant.
2. Add carrots, zucchini, lentils, and vegetable broth.
3. Season with cumin, salt, and pepper. Simmer until lentils are tender.
4. Serve hot with a sprinkle of fresh herbs.

Nutrition Information:

- Calories: 250
- Protein: 15g
- Carbohydrates: 45g
- Fat: 2g
- Fiber: 12g
- Portion Size: 1 cup

Grilled Chicken Salad

Ingredients:

- 2 boneless, skinless chicken breasts
- 6 cups mixed greens
- 1 cup cherry tomatoes, halved
- 1 cucumber, sliced
- 1/4 cup feta cheese, crumbled

- Balsamic vinaigrette dressing

Instructions:

1. Grill chicken breasts until cooked through.

2. Slice chicken into strips.

3. Toss mixed greens, cherry tomatoes, cucumber, and feta.

4. Top with grilled chicken and drizzle with balsamic vinaigrette.

Nutrition Information:

- Calories: 320
- Protein: 30g
- Carbohydrates: 15g
- Fat: 15g
- Fiber: 5g
- Portion Size: 2 cups

Quinoa and Black Bean Bowl

Ingredients:

- 1 cup cooked quinoa
- 1 can black beans, drained and rinsed

- 1 red bell pepper, diced

- 1 avocado, sliced

- Fresh cilantro, chopped

- Lime wedges

Instructions:

1. Mix quinoa, black beans, and diced bell pepper.

2. Divide into bowls and top with avocado slices.

3. Garnish with cilantro and serve with lime wedges.

Nutrition Information:

- Calories: 380

- Protein: 15g

- Carbohydrates: 50g

- Fat: 15g

- Fiber: 15g

- Portion Size: 1.5 cups

Salmon and Asparagus Parcels

Ingredients:

- 4 salmon fillets

- 1 bunch asparagus, trimmed

- 2 lemons, sliced

- Fresh dill

- Salt and pepper to taste

Instructions:

1. Preheat oven to 400°F (200°C).

2. Season salmon with salt and pepper.

3. Create parcels with salmon, asparagus, lemon slices, and dill.

4. Bake for 15-20 minutes until salmon is cooked.

Nutrition Information:

- Calories: 320

- Protein: 30g

- Carbohydrates: 10g

- Fat: 20g

- Fiber: 5g

- Portion Size: 1 parcel

Turkey and Vegetable Stir-Fry

Ingredients:

- 1 lb ground turkey

- 2 cups broccoli florets
- 1 bell pepper, sliced
- 1 cup snap peas
- 3 tablespoons soy sauce
- 1 tablespoon sesame oil

Instructions:

1. Brown turkey in a wok or skillet.
2. Add vegetables and stir-fry until tender-crisp.
3. Mix in soy sauce and sesame oil.
4. Serve over brown rice or quinoa.

Nutrition Information:

- Calories: 280
- Protein: 25g
- Carbohydrates: 15g
- Fat: 15g
- Fiber: 5g
- Portion Size: 1.5 cups

Caprese Salad with Balsamic Glaze

Ingredients:

- 4 large tomatoes, sliced
- 1 lb fresh mozzarella, sliced
- Fresh basil leaves
- Balsamic glaze
- Salt and pepper to taste

Instructions:

1. Arrange tomato and mozzarella slices on a platter.
2. Tuck in fresh basil leaves.
3. Drizzle with balsamic glaze.
4. Season with salt and pepper.

Nutrition Information:

- Calories: 280
- Protein: 20g
- Carbohydrates: 10g
- Fat: 20g
- Fiber: 2g
- Portion Size: 1 cup

Chickpea and Spinach Curry

Ingredients:

- 2 cans chickpeas, drained
- 1 onion, finely chopped
- 3 cloves garlic, minced
- 1 can diced tomatoes
- 2 cups fresh spinach
- 2 tablespoons curry powder

Instructions:

1. Sauté onions and garlic until golden.
2. Add chickpeas, tomatoes, and curry powder.
3. Simmer until flavors meld.
4. Stir in fresh spinach until wilted.

Nutrition Information:

- Calories: 320
- Protein: 18g
- Carbohydrates: 45g
- Fat: 8g
- Fiber: 15g
- Portion Size: 1.5 cups

Shrimp and Quinoa Salad

Ingredients:

- 1 lb shrimp, peeled and deveined
- 1 cup cooked quinoa
- 1 cup cherry tomatoes, halved
- 1 cucumber, diced
- 1/4 cup feta cheese, crumbled
- Lemon vinaigrette dressing

Instructions:

1. Grill or sauté shrimp until pink and opaque.
2. Combine cooked quinoa, cherry tomatoes, cucumber, and feta.
3. Top with shrimp and drizzle with lemon vinaigrette.

Nutrition Information:

- Calories: 290
- Protein: 25g
- Carbohydrates: 25g
- Fat: 10g
- Fiber: 4g
- Portion Size: 1.5 cups

Sweet Potato and Kale Salad

Ingredients:

- 2 sweet potatoes, diced
- 4 cups kale, chopped
- 1/2 cup dried cranberries
- 1/4 cup sunflower seeds
- Dijon mustard dressing

Instructions:

1. Roast sweet potatoes until tender.
2. Massage kale with dressing.
3. Toss sweet potatoes, kale, cranberries, and sunflower seeds.

Nutrition Information:

- Calories: 280
- Protein: 8g
- Carbohydrates: 45g
- Fat: 10g
- Fiber: 8g
- Portion Size: 2 cups

Ratatouille with Brown Rice

Ingredients:

- 1 eggplant, diced
- 2 zucchinis, sliced
- 1 bell pepper, diced
- 1 onion, chopped
- 2 cloves garlic, minced
- 1 can diced tomatoes
- Fresh thyme and rosemary
- Cooked brown rice

Instructions:

1. Sauté onion and garlic until softened.
2. Add eggplant, zucchini, bell pepper, and diced tomatoes.
3. Simmer until vegetables are tender.
4. Season with thyme and rosemary. Serve over brown rice.

Nutrition Information:

- Calories: 250
- Protein: 6g

- Carbohydrates: 55g
- Fat: 2g
- Fiber: 12g
- Portion Size: 1.5 cups

Tofu and Broccoli Stir-Fry

Ingredients:

- 1 block extra-firm tofu, cubed
- 3 cups broccoli florets
- 1 bell pepper, sliced
- 2 tablespoons soy sauce
- 1 tablespoon hoisin sauce

Instructions:

1. Press tofu to remove excess moisture.
2. Stir-fry tofu until golden.
3. Add broccoli and bell pepper.
4. Drizzle with soy sauce and hoisin. Serve over quinoa.

Nutrition Information:

- Calories: 290
- Protein: 18g

- Carbohydrates: 30g

- Fat: 14g

- Fiber: 8g

- Portion Size: 1.5 cups

Caesar Salad with Grilled Chicken

Ingredients:

- 2 boneless, skinless chicken breasts

- Romaine lettuce, chopped

- Croutons

- Parmesan cheese, shaved

- Caesar dressing

Instructions:

1. Grill chicken breasts until cooked.

2. Slice chicken and toss with lettuce, croutons, and Parmesan.

3. Drizzle with Caesar dressing.

Nutrition Information:

- Calories: 350

- Protein: 30g

- Carbohydrates: 15g

- Fat: 18g

- Fiber: 4g

- Portion Size: 2 cups

Mediterranean Chickpea Wrap

Ingredients:

- 1 can chickpeas, mashed

- 1 cucumber, sliced

- 1 tomato, diced

- Kalamata olives, sliced

- Feta cheese, crumbled

- Whole grain wraps

Instructions:

1. Spread mashed chickpeas on wraps.

2. Add cucumber, tomato, olives, and feta.

3. Roll tightly and slice in half.

Nutrition Information:

- Calories: 320

- Protein: 15g

- Carbohydrates: 45g
- Fat: 10g
- Fiber: 10g
- Portion Size: 1 wrap

Zucchini Noodles with Pesto

Ingredients:

- 4 medium zucchinis, spiralized
- Cherry tomatoes, halved
- Pesto sauce
- Pine nuts, toasted

Instructions:

1. Spiralize zucchinis into noodles.
2. Toss with cherry tomatoes and pesto.
3. Top with toasted pine nuts.

Nutrition Information:

- Calories: 260
- Protein: 8g
- Carbohydrates: 20g
- Fat: 18g

- Fiber: 6g

- Portion Size: 1.5 cups

Spinach and Mushroom Quesadilla

Ingredients:

- Whole grain tortillas

- 2 cups spinach, chopped

- 1 cup mushrooms, sliced

- 1 cup shredded cheese (your choice)

- Salsa for dipping

Instructions:

1. Lay out tortillas and layer with spinach, mushrooms, and cheese.

2. Top with another tortilla.

3. Cook on a griddle until cheese melts. Slice into wedges.

Nutrition Information:

- Calories: 280

- Protein: 15g

- Carbohydrates: 30g

- Fat: 12g
- Fiber: 6g
- Portion Size: 1 quesadilla

Chapter 4: Dinner Recipes

Welcome to Chapter 4 of our "Complete Renal Diet Cookbook" where we explore delightful dinner recipes designed for renal health. Each dish is thoughtfully crafted with flavorful ingredients to provide both satisfaction and nourishment. Let's embark on a culinary journey that supports your well-being.

Baked Cod with Lemon and Herbs

Ingredients:

- 4 cod fillets
- 2 tablespoons olive oil
- 1 lemon (zested and juiced)
- 2 cloves garlic (minced)
- 1 tablespoon fresh parsley (chopped)
- Salt and pepper to taste

Instructions:

1. Preheat the oven to 375°F (190°C).
2. Place cod fillets in a baking dish.

3. In a bowl, mix olive oil, lemon zest, lemon juice, minced garlic, chopped parsley, salt, and pepper.

4. Pour the mixture over the cod.

5. Bake for 15-20 minutes or until the fish flakes easily.

6. Serve with a side of steamed vegetables.

Nutrition Information:

1. Calories: 250

2. Protein: 30g

3. Carbohydrates: 2g

4. Fat: 12g

5. Fiber: 0.5g

6. Portion Size: 1 fillet

Eggplant Parmesan

Ingredients:

- 2 large eggplants (sliced)

- 2 cups marinara sauce

- 1 cup mozzarella cheese (shredded)

- 1/2 cup Parmesan cheese (grated)

- 1/4 cup fresh basil (chopped)

- Salt and pepper to taste

Instructions:

1. Preheat the oven to 400°F (200°C).
2. Salt eggplant slices and let them sit for 30 minutes, then pat dry.
3. Layer eggplant slices, marinara sauce, mozzarella, and Parmesan in a baking dish.
4. Repeat the layers and finish with cheese on top.
5. Bake for 25-30 minutes until golden and bubbly.
6. Garnish with fresh basil before serving.

Nutrition Information:

- Calories: 280
- Protein: 10g
- Carbohydrates: 15g
- Fat: 20g
- Fiber: 7g
- Portion Size: 1 cup

Chicken and Vegetable Skewers

Ingredients:

- 1 lb chicken breast (cubed)
- 2 bell peppers (cut into chunks)

- 1 red onion (cut into chunks)

- 2 tablespoons olive oil

- 1 teaspoon paprika

- 1 teaspoon garlic powder

- Salt and pepper to taste

Instructions:

1. Preheat the grill or grill pan.
2. In a bowl, mix chicken, bell peppers, red onion, olive oil, paprika, garlic powder, salt, and pepper.
3. Thread onto skewers, alternating between chicken and vegetables.
4. Grill for 10-15 minutes, turning occasionally until chicken is cooked through.
5. Serve with a side of quinoa or brown rice.

Nutrition Information:

- Calories: 320

- Protein: 25g

- Carbohydrates: 10g

- Fat: 18g

- Fiber: 3g

- Portion Size: 2 skewers

Quinoa-Stuffed Bell Peppers

Ingredients:

- 4 bell peppers (halved and seeds removed)
- 1 cup cooked quinoa
- 1 can black beans (drained and rinsed)
- 1 cup corn kernels
- 1 cup cherry tomatoes (halved)
- 1 teaspoon cumin
- 1 teaspoon chili powder
- Salt and pepper to taste

Instructions:

1. Preheat the oven to 375°F (190°C).
2. In a bowl, combine quinoa, black beans, corn, cherry tomatoes, cumin, chili powder, salt, and pepper.
3. Stuff each bell pepper half with the quinoa mixture.
4. Bake for 20-25 minutes until peppers are tender.
5. Garnish with fresh cilantro before serving.

Nutrition Information:

- Calories: 280
- Protein: 12g
- Carbohydrates: 50g
- Fat: 4g
- Fiber: 10g
- Portion Size: 2 pepper halves

Teriyaki Salmon with Vegetables

Ingredients:

- 4 salmon fillets
- 1/4 cup teriyaki sauce
- 2 tablespoons soy sauce
- 1 tablespoon honey
- 1 teaspoon ginger (minced)
- 2 cups broccoli florets
- 1 red bell pepper (sliced)
- 1 carrot (julienned)

Instructions:

1. Preheat the oven to 400°F (200°C).

2. In a bowl, mix teriyaki sauce, soy sauce, honey, and minced ginger.

3. Place salmon fillets on a baking sheet, surround with broccoli, red bell pepper, and carrot.

4. Brush salmon and vegetables with the teriyaki mixture.

5. Bake for 15-20 minutes or until salmon is cooked through.

6. Serve over brown rice.

Nutrition Information:

- Calories: 340
- Protein: 28g
- Carbohydrates: 25g
- Fat: 15g
- Fiber: 5g
- Portion Size: 1 fillet with vegetables

Turkey and Quinoa Meatballs

Ingredients:

- 1 lb ground turkey
- 1 cup cooked quinoa

- 1/4 cup breadcrumbs
- 1/4 cup grated Parmesan cheese
- 1 egg
- 2 cloves garlic (minced)
- 1 teaspoon Italian seasoning
- Salt and pepper to taste

Instructions:

1. Preheat the oven to 375°F (190°C).
2. In a bowl, combine ground turkey, cooked quinoa, breadcrumbs, Parmesan cheese, egg, minced garlic, Italian seasoning, salt, and pepper.
3. Form the mixture into meatballs and place on a baking sheet.
4. Bake for 20-25 minutes or until cooked through.
5. Serve with a side of steamed vegetables.

Nutrition Information:

- Calories: 240
- Protein: 20g
- Carbohydrates: 15g
- Fat: 10g

- Fiber: 2g
- Portion Size: 4 meatballs

Vegetable and Lentil Curry

Ingredients:

- 1 cup dry lentils (rinsed)
- 2 cups mixed vegetables (e.g., cauliflower, carrots, peas)
- 1 onion (chopped)
- 2 tomatoes (chopped)
- 1 can coconut milk
- 2 tablespoons curry powder
- 1 teaspoon turmeric
- Salt and pepper to taste

Instructions:

1. In a pot, combine lentils, mixed vegetables, chopped onion, tomatoes, coconut milk, curry powder, turmeric, salt, and pepper.
2. Bring to a boil, then simmer until lentils are tender.
3. Serve over brown rice.

Nutrition Information:

- Calories: 300
- Protein: 15g
- Carbohydrates: 40g
- Fat: 10g
- Fiber: 15g
- Portion Size: 1 cup

Grilled Swordfish with Mango Salsa

Ingredients:

- 4 swordfish steaks
- 1 mango (peeled and diced)
- 1/2 red onion (finely chopped)
- 1 jalapeño (seeded and minced)
- 1/4 cup cilantro (chopped)
- Juice of 1 lime
- Salt and pepper to taste

Instructions:

1. Preheat the grill.
2. Season swordfish steaks with salt and pepper.

3. Grill for 4-5 minutes per side or until cooked through.

4. In a bowl, combine diced mango, chopped red onion, minced jalapeño, cilantro, lime juice, salt, and pepper.

5. Serve swordfish topped with mango salsa.

Nutrition Information:

- Calories: 320

- Protein: 30g

- Carbohydrates: 15g

- Fat: 15g

- Fiber: 3g

- Portion Size: 1 steak with salsa

Spinach and Ricotta Stuffed Chicken Breast

Ingredients:

- 4 chicken breasts

- 2 cups fresh spinach (chopped)

- 1 cup ricotta cheese

- 1/4 cup grated Parmesan cheese
- 2 cloves garlic (minced)
- 1 teaspoon dried oregano
- Salt and pepper to taste

Instructions:

1. Preheat the oven to 375°F (190°C).
2. In a bowl, mix chopped spinach, ricotta cheese, grated Parmesan, minced garlic, dried oregano, salt, and pepper.
3. Cut a pocket into each chicken breast and stuff with the spinach and ricotta mixture.
4. Bake for 25-30 minutes or until chicken is cooked through.
5. Serve with a side of roasted vegetables.

Nutrition Information:

- Calories: 280
- Protein: 35g
- Carbohydrates: 5g
- Fat: 12g
- Fiber: 2g

- Portion Size: 1 stuffed chicken breast

Portobello Mushroom Steaks

Ingredients:

- 4 large portobello mushrooms
- 1/4 cup balsamic vinegar
- 2 tablespoons olive oil
- 2 cloves garlic (minced)
- 1 teaspoon dried thyme
- Salt and pepper to taste

Instructions:

1. Preheat the oven to 400°F (200°C).
2. Clean portobello mushrooms and remove stems.
3. In a bowl, mix balsamic vinegar, olive oil, minced garlic, dried thyme, salt, and pepper.
4. Brush the mixture onto both sides of each mushroom.
5. Roast for 20-25 minutes or until mushrooms are tender.
6. Serve as a main dish or alongside a protein.

Nutrition Information:

- Calories: 120
- Protein: 5g
- Carbohydrates: 10g
- Fat: 8g
- Fiber: 3g
- Portion Size: 1 mushroom

Pesto Zoodles with Cherry Tomatoes

Ingredients:

- 4 zucchinis (spiralized into noodles)
- 1 cup cherry tomatoes (halved)
- 1/4 cup pesto sauce
- 2 tablespoons pine nuts
- 1/4 cup grated Parmesan cheese
- Salt and pepper to taste

Instructions:

1. In a pan, sauté zucchini noodles until just tender.

2. Toss with cherry tomatoes, pesto sauce, pine nuts, Parmesan, salt, and pepper.

3. Cook for an additional 2-3 minutes.

4. Serve immediately.

Nutrition Information:

- Calories: 180
- Protein: 5g
- Carbohydrates: 12g
- Fat: 14g
- Fiber: 4g
- Portion Size: 1 cup

Black Bean and Vegetable Stir-Fry

Ingredients:

- 2 cups black beans (cooked)
- 2 cups mixed vegetables (e.g., broccoli, bell peppers, snap peas)
- 2 tablespoons soy sauce
- 1 tablespoon sesame oil
- 1 tablespoon rice vinegar
- 1 teaspoon ginger (minced)

- 2 cloves garlic (minced)
- 1 tablespoon sesame seeds
- Green onions for garnish

Instructions:

1. In a wok or pan, stir-fry mixed vegetables until crisp-tender.
2. Add black beans, soy sauce, sesame oil, rice vinegar, minced ginger, and minced garlic.
3. Stir-fry for an additional 3-5 minutes.
4. Sprinkle with sesame seeds and garnish with green onions.
5. Serve over brown rice.

Nutrition Information:

- Calories: 280
- Protein: 15g
- Carbohydrates: 40g
- Fat: 8g
- Fiber: 10g
- Portion Size: 1 cup

Baked Chicken with Rosemary

Ingredients:

- 4 chicken thighs
- 2 tablespoons olive oil
- 1 tablespoon fresh rosemary (chopped)
- 2 cloves garlic (minced)
- Salt and pepper to taste

Instructions:

1. Preheat the oven to 400°F (200°C).
2. Rub chicken thighs with olive oil, chopped rosemary, minced garlic, salt, and pepper.
3. Place on a baking sheet and bake for 30-35 minutes or until chicken is golden and cooked through.
4. Serve with a side of roasted sweet potatoes.

Nutrition Information:

- Calories: 320
- Protein: 25g
- Carbohydrates: 0g
- Fat: 24g
- Fiber: 0g

- Portion Size: 1 chicken thigh

Cauliflower and Chickpea Curry

Ingredients:

- 1 cauliflower (cut into florets)
- 1 can chickpeas (drained and rinsed)
- 1 onion (chopped)
- 2 tomatoes (chopped)
- 1 can coconut milk
- 2 tablespoons curry powder
- 1 teaspoon turmeric
- Salt and pepper to taste

Instructions:

1. In a pot, combine cauliflower, chickpeas, chopped onion, tomatoes, coconut milk, curry powder, turmeric, salt, and pepper.
2. Bring to a boil, then simmer until cauliflower is tender.
3. Serve over quinoa.

Nutrition Information:

- Calories: 280
- Protein: 10g
- Carbohydrates: 35g
- Fat: 12g
- Fiber: 10g
- Portion Size: 1 cup

Lemon Garlic Shrimp Skewers

Ingredients:

- 1 lb shrimp (peeled and deveined)
- 2 tablespoons olive oil
- 2 cloves garlic (minced)
- Zest and juice of 1 lemon
- 1 teaspoon dried oregano
- Salt and pepper to taste

Instructions:

1. Preheat the grill or grill pan.
2. In a bowl, mix shrimp, olive oil, minced garlic, lemon zest, lemon juice, dried oregano, salt, and pepper.

3. Thread shrimp onto skewers.

4. Grill for 2-3 minutes per side or until shrimp are opaque.

5. Serve with a side of quinoa or a green salad.

Nutrition Information:

- Calories: 200
- Protein: 25g
- Carbohydrates: 2g
- Fat: 10g
- Fiber: 0g
- Portion Size: 1 cup

Chapter 5: Snacks and Appetizers

Indulge in a delightful array of snacks and appetizers designed to tantalize your taste buds while keeping your health in mind. From savory dips to crunchy delights, each recipe is crafted for both flavor and nutrition. Elevate your snacking experience with these enticing options that cater to your cravings without compromising on wellness.

Hummus with Veggie Sticks

Ingredients:

- 1 can chickpeas, drained and rinsed
- 2 cloves garlic, minced
- 1/4 cup tahini
- 3 tablespoons olive oil
- 2 tablespoons lemon juice
- Salt and pepper to taste
- Assorted vegetable sticks (carrots, cucumber, bell peppers)

Instructions:

1. Blend chickpeas, garlic, tahini, olive oil, and lemon juice until smooth.
2. Season with salt and pepper to taste.
3. Serve with a colorful assortment of vegetable sticks.

Nutrition Information:

- Calories: 120
- Protein: 4g
- Carbohydrates: 12g
- Fat: 7g
- Fiber: 3g
- Portion Size: 2 tablespoons hummus with veggies

Guacamole with Whole Grain Chips

Ingredients:

- 3 ripe avocados
- 1 tomato, diced
- 1/4 cup red onion, finely chopped
- 1 clove garlic, minced
- 2 tablespoons fresh cilantro, chopped
- Lime juice, to taste

- Whole grain tortilla chips

Instructions:

1. Mash avocados and mix with tomato, red onion, garlic, and cilantro.

2. Add lime juice and salt to taste.

3. Serve with whole grain tortilla chips.

Nutrition Information:

- Calories: 160

- Protein: 3g

- Carbohydrates: 10g

- Fat: 14g

- Fiber: 6g

- Portion Size: 1/2 cup guacamole with chips

Greek Yogurt and Cucumber Dip

Ingredients:

- 1 cup Greek yogurt

- 1 cucumber, finely diced

- 2 tablespoons fresh dill, chopped

- 1 clove garlic, minced

- Salt and pepper to taste

Instructions:

1. Combine Greek yogurt, cucumber, dill, and garlic.

2. Season with salt and pepper to taste.

3. Refrigerate before serving with your favorite dippables.

Nutrition Information:

- Calories: 80

- Protein: 10g

- Carbohydrates: 8g

- Fat: 1g

- Fiber: 1g

- Portion Size: 1/4 cup dip

Mixed Nuts and Seeds

Ingredients:

- 1 cup mixed nuts (almonds, walnuts, cashews)

- 2 tablespoons pumpkin seeds

- 2 tablespoons sunflower seeds

- 1 tablespoon honey

- 1/2 teaspoon cinnamon

- Pinch of sea salt

Instructions:

1. Roast mixed nuts and seeds in a pan until golden.

2. Drizzle honey, sprinkle cinnamon, and add a pinch of sea salt.

3. Toss until evenly coated and let it cool before serving.

Nutrition Information:

- Calories: 200

- Protein: 6g

- Carbohydrates: 10g

- Fat: 16g

- Fiber: 3g

- Portion Size: 1/4 cup serving

Stuffed Grape Leaves

Ingredients:

- Grape leaves, jarred or fresh

- 1 cup cooked quinoa

- 1/4 cup pine nuts

- 1/4 cup fresh parsley, chopped

- Lemon juice, to taste

- Greek yogurt for dipping

Instructions:

1. Mix cooked quinoa, pine nuts, parsley, and lemon juice.

2. Place a spoonful on a grape leaf and roll tightly.

3. Serve with a side of Greek yogurt.

Nutrition Information:

- Calories: 150

- Protein: 4g

- Carbohydrates: 20g

- Fat: 6g

- Fiber: 3g

- Portion Size: 2 stuffed grape leaves

Baked Sweet Potato Fries

Ingredients:

- 2 large sweet potatoes, cut into fries

- 1 tablespoon olive oil

- 1 teaspoon paprika

- 1/2 teaspoon garlic powder

- Salt and pepper to taste

Instructions:

1. Toss sweet potato fries in olive oil and seasonings.

2. Arrange on a baking sheet and bake until crispy.

3. Serve hot with your preferred dipping sauce.

Nutrition Information:

- Calories: 120

- Protein: 2g

- Carbohydrates: 25g

- Fat: 2g

- Fiber: 4g

- Portion Size: 1 cup serving

Edamame with Sea Salt

Ingredients:

- 2 cups edamame, shelled

- Sea salt, to taste

Instructions:

1. Boil or steam edamame until tender.

2. Sprinkle with sea salt and toss to coat.

3. Enjoy these delightful, protein-packed green bites.

Nutrition Information:

- Calories: 150

- Protein: 17g

- Carbohydrates: 13g

- Fat: 8g

- Fiber: 8g

- Portion Size: 1 cup serving

Caprese Skewers

Ingredients:

- Cherry tomatoes

- Fresh mozzarella balls

- Fresh basil leaves

- Balsamic glaze

Instructions:

1. Thread a tomato, mozzarella ball, and basil leaf onto small skewers.

2. Arrange on a platter and drizzle with balsamic glaze.

3. A classic combination for a light and flavorful snack.

Nutrition Information:

- Calories: 120

- Protein: 8g

- Carbohydrates: 5g

- Fat: 8g

- Fiber: 1g

- Portion Size: 3 skewers

Roasted Chickpeas

Ingredients:

- 1 can chickpeas, drained and rinsed

- 1 tablespoon olive oil

- 1 teaspoon cumin

- 1/2 teaspoon smoked paprika

- Salt to taste

Instructions:

1. Toss chickpeas in olive oil, cumin, paprika, and salt.
2. Roast in the oven until crispy.
3. A crunchy and flavorful protein-packed snack.

Nutrition Information:

- Calories: 160
- Protein: 6g
- Carbohydrates: 22g
- Fat: 6g
- Fiber: 6g
- Portion Size: 1/2 cup serving

Avocado Bruschetta

Ingredients:

- 2 ripe avocados, diced
- 1 cup cherry tomatoes, halved
- 1/4 cup red onion, finely chopped
- 2 tablespoons fresh basil, chopped
- 1 tablespoon balsamic vinegar
- Salt and pepper to taste
- Whole grain baguette slices

Instructions:

1. Combine avocados, cherry tomatoes, red onion, basil, and balsamic vinegar.
2. Season with salt and pepper to taste.
3. Serve the mixture on whole grain baguette slices.

Nutrition Information:

- Calories: 180
- Protein: 4g
- Carbohydrates: 22g
- Fat: 10g
- Fiber: 7g
- Portion Size: 2 slices with topping

Spicy Tuna Lettuce Wraps

Ingredients:

- 1 can tuna in water, drained
- 1 tablespoon mayonnaise
- Sriracha sauce, to taste
- Butter lettuce leaves

Instructions:

1. Mix tuna with mayonnaise and Sriracha.
2. Spoon the mixture onto butter lettuce leaves.
3. A satisfying and spicy low-carb option.

Nutrition Information:

- Calories: 140
- Protein: 18g
- Carbohydrates: 2g
- Fat: 7g
- Fiber: 1g
- Portion Size: 2 lettuce wraps

Cottage Cheese and Tomato Slices

Ingredients:

- Low-fat cottage cheese
- Ripe tomatoes, sliced
- Fresh basil leaves
- Balsamic glaze

Instructions:

1. Arrange cottage cheese and tomato slices on a plate.

2. Garnish with fresh basil and drizzle with balsamic glaze.

3. A simple and protein-packed snack.

Nutrition Information:

- Calories: 120
- Protein: 14g
- Carbohydrates: 8g
- Fat: 3g
- Fiber: 1g
- Portion Size: 1 cup serving

Sliced Apple with Almond Butter

Ingredients:

- 2 medium apples, sliced
- Almond butter

Instructions:

1. Slice apples into thin wedges.

2. Serve with a side of almond butter for dipping.

3. A delightful combination of sweetness and nuttiness.

Nutrition Information:

- Calories: 180
- Protein: 4g
- Carbohydrates: 26g
- Fat: 9g
- Fiber: 6g
- Portion Size: 1 medium apple with 2 tablespoons almond butter

Veggie Spring Rolls

Ingredients:

- Rice paper wrappers
- Shredded cabbage
- Carrots, julienned
- Cucumber, julienned
- Fresh mint leaves
- Dipping sauce of choice

Instructions:

1. Soften rice paper wrappers in warm water.
2. Fill with shredded cabbage, carrots, cucumber, and mint.

3. Roll tightly and serve with your favorite dipping sauce.

Nutrition Information:

- Calories: 100
- Protein: 2g
- Carbohydrates: 22g
- Fat: 0g
- Fiber: 3g
- Portion Size: 2 spring rolls

Beetroot and Goat Cheese Crostini

Ingredients:

- Baguette slices, toasted
- Roasted beetroot, thinly sliced
- Goat cheese
- Honey for drizzling
- Fresh thyme leaves

Instructions:

1. Top toasted baguette slices with roasted beetroot.

2. Add a dollop of goat cheese on each slice.

3. Drizzle with honey and garnish with fresh thyme.

Nutrition Information:

- Calories: 120

- Protein: 4g

- Carbohydrates: 15g

- Fat: 5g

- Fiber: 2g

- Portion Size: 3 crostini

Chapter 6: Desserts

Indulge your taste buds with the delectable delights awaiting you in this dessert chapter. Each recipe is crafted to satisfy your sweet cravings while adhering to the principles of a wholesome renal diet. Let the richness of flavors and the variety of textures captivate your senses. From fruity parfaits to creamy tarts, these desserts are a delightful finale to your renal-friendly meals.

Berry and Yogurt Parfait

Ingredients:

- 1 cup Greek yogurt
- 1/2 cup mixed berries (strawberries, blueberries, raspberries)
- 1 tablespoon honey
- Granola for topping

Instructions:

1. In a glass or bowl, layer Greek yogurt.
2. Add a layer of mixed berries.

3. Drizzle with honey.

4. Repeat layers.

5. Top with granola.

6. Serve chilled.

Nutrition Information:

- Calories: 250

- Protein: 15g

- Carbohydrates: 35g

- Fat: 8g

- Fiber: 5g

- Portion Size: 1 serving

Mango Sorbet

Ingredients:

- 2 ripe mangoes, peeled and diced

- 1/4 cup honey

- 1 tablespoon lime juice

Instructions:

1. Blend diced mangoes until smooth.

2. Add honey and lime juice; blend again.

3. Pour into a container and freeze for 4-6 hours.

4. Scoop and enjoy.

Nutrition Information:

- Calories: 180

- Protein: 2g

- Carbohydrates: 45g

- Fat: 0g

- Fiber: 3g

- Portion Size: 1 serving

Dark Chocolate Avocado Mousse

Ingredients:

- 2 ripe avocados

- 1/4 cup cocoa powder

- 1/4 cup maple syrup

- 1 teaspoon vanilla extract

Instructions:

1. Blend avocados until creamy.

2. Add cocoa powder, maple syrup, and vanilla extract; blend.

3. Refrigerate for 2 hours.

4. Serve chilled.

Nutrition Information:

- Calories: 200

- Protein: 3g

- Carbohydrates: 20g

- Fat: 15g

- Fiber: 7g

- Portion Size: 1 serving

Baked Apple with Cinnamon

Ingredients:

- 2 apples, cored and sliced

- 1 tablespoon cinnamon

- 1 tablespoon honey

- 1/4 cup chopped walnuts

Instructions:

1. Preheat oven to 350°F (175°C).

2. Place apple slices in a baking dish.

3. Sprinkle with cinnamon and drizzle honey.

4. Bake for 20-25 minutes until tender.

5. Top with chopped walnuts before serving.

Nutrition Information:

- Calories: 160

- Protein: 2g

- Carbohydrates: 30g

- Fat: 5g

- Fiber: 6g

- Portion Size: 1 serving

Chia Seed Pudding with Berries

Ingredients:

- 2 tablespoons chia seeds

- 1 cup almond milk

- 1/2 teaspoon vanilla extract

- Mixed berries for topping

Instructions:

1. Mix chia seeds, almond milk, and vanilla extract.

2. Refrigerate for at least 4 hours or overnight.

3. Top with mixed berries before serving.

Nutrition Information:

- Calories: 120
- Protein: 4g
- Carbohydrates: 15g
- Fat: 6g
- Fiber: 8g
- Portion Size: 1 serving

Almond and Coconut Energy Bites

Ingredients:

- 1 cup almonds
- 1/2 cup shredded coconut
- 1/4 cup honey
- 1/2 teaspoon vanilla extract

Instructions:

1. Blend almonds and shredded coconut.
2. Add honey and vanilla extract; mix well.
3. Roll into bite-sized balls.
4. Refrigerate for 1 hour before serving.

Nutrition Information:

- Calories: 180
- Protein: 5g
- Carbohydrates: 15g
- Fat: 12g
- Fiber: 3g
- Portion Size: 1 serving

Greek Yogurt and Honey Tart

Ingredients:

- 1 pre-made whole-grain tart shell
- 1 1/2 cups Greek yogurt
- 1/4 cup honey
- Fresh berries for topping

Instructions:

1. Spread Greek yogurt evenly in the tart shell.
2. Drizzle honey over the yogurt.
3. Top with fresh berries.
4. Refrigerate for 1 hour before serving.

Nutrition Information:

- Calories: 220
- Protein: 10g
- Carbohydrates: 30g
- Fat: 8g
- Fiber: 2g
- Portion Size: 1 serving

Watermelon Granita

Ingredients:

- 4 cups seedless watermelon, cubed
- 2 tablespoons fresh lime juice
- 2 tablespoons mint leaves, chopped

Instructions:

1. Blend watermelon until smooth.
2. Stir in lime juice and mint.
3. Pour into a shallow dish and freeze.
4. Scrape with a fork before serving.

Nutrition Information:

- Calories: 90
- Protein: 1g
- Carbohydrates: 22g
- Fat: 0g
- Fiber: 1g
- Portion Size: 1 serving

Poached Pears in Red Wine

Ingredients:

- 4 ripe pears, peeled and halved
- 1 bottle red wine
- 1/2 cup honey
- 1 cinnamon stick

Instructions:

1. In a saucepan, combine red wine, honey, and cinnamon.
2. Add pears and simmer until tender.
3. Serve pears with reduced wine sauce.

Nutrition Information:

- Calories: 180
- Protein: 1g
- Carbohydrates: 40g
- Fat: 0g
- Fiber: 5g
- Portion Size: 1 serving

Pistachio and Cranberry Bark

Ingredients:

- 1 cup dark chocolate, melted
- 1/2 cup pistachios, chopped
- 1/4 cup dried cranberries

Instructions:

1. Line a tray with parchment paper.
2. Pour melted chocolate onto the paper.
3. Sprinkle with pistachios and cranberries.
4. Refrigerate until set, then break into pieces.

Nutrition Information:

- Calories: 160
- Protein: 3g
- Carbohydrates: 20g
- Fat: 8g
- Fiber: 2g
- Portion Size: 1 serving

Pumpkin Pie Smoothie Bowl

Ingredients:

- 1 cup pumpkin puree
- 1 frozen banana
- 1/2 cup almond milk
- 1/2 teaspoon pumpkin spice
- Toppings: granola, pumpkin seeds

Instructions:

1. Blend pumpkin puree, frozen banana, almond milk, and pumpkin spice until smooth.
2. Pour into a bowl and add granola and pumpkin seeds on top.

Nutrition Information:

- Calories: 220
- Protein: 5g
- Carbohydrates: 40g
- Fat: 6g
- Fiber: 8g
- Portion Size: 1 serving

Blueberry Oat Bars

Ingredients:

- 2 cups rolled oats
- 1 cup blueberries
- 1/4 cup honey
- 1/4 cup almond butter

Instructions:

1. Mix rolled oats, blueberries, honey, and almond butter.
2. Press into a baking dish and refrigerate for 2 hours.
3. Cut into bars before serving.

Nutrition Information:

- Calories: 180
- Protein: 5g
- Carbohydrates: 30g
- Fat: 6g
- Fiber: 4g
- Portion Size: 1 serving

Peach and Berry Cobbler

Ingredients:

- 2 cups sliced peaches
- 1 cup mixed berries
- 1 tablespoon maple syrup
- Topping: oat crumble

Instructions:

1. Preheat oven to 350°F (175°C).
2. Mix peaches, berries, and maple syrup.
3. Transfer to a baking dish, top with oat crumble.
4. Bake for 30-35 minutes.

Nutrition Information:

- Calories: 160
- Protein: 3g
- Carbohydrates: 35g
- Fat: 2g
- Fiber: 5g
- Portion Size: 1 serving

Lemon Poppy Seed Muffins

Ingredients:

- 2 cups almond flour
- 1/4 cup coconut flour
- 1/4 cup poppy seeds
- 1/2 teaspoon baking soda
- 3 eggs
- 1/4 cup coconut oil
- Zest and juice of 2 lemons

Instructions:

1. Mix almond flour, coconut flour, poppy seeds, and baking soda.

2. In a separate bowl, whisk eggs, coconut oil, lemon zest, and juice.

3. Combine wet and dry ingredients.

4. Spoon into muffin cups and bake for 20-25 minutes.

Nutrition Information:

- Calories: 220
- Protein: 8g
- Carbohydrates: 10g
- Fat: 18g
- Fiber: 4g
- Portion Size: 1 muffin

Banana Ice Cream

Ingredients:

- 4 ripe bananas, frozen
- 1/4 cup almond milk
- Toppings: sliced almonds, dark chocolate chips

Instructions:

1. Blend frozen bananas and almond milk until creamy.

2. Serve immediately with sliced almonds and dark chocolate chips.

Nutrition Information:

- Calories: 150
- Protein: 3g
- Carbohydrates: 35g
- Fat: 2g
- Fiber: 5g
- Portion Size: 1 serving

Chapter 7: Smoothies

Embark on a journey of vibrant flavors and wholesome nutrition with our collection of delightful smoothie recipes in Chapter 7. Each blend is crafted to tantalize your taste buds while nourishing your body. From the invigorating Green Detox Smoothie to the luscious Watermelon Mint Smoothie, discover a symphony of ingredients that promise a refreshing twist to your daily routine.

Green Detox Smoothie

Ingredients:

- 1 cup spinach
- 1/2 cucumber, peeled
- 1/2 green apple, cored
- 1/2 lemon, juiced
- 1 cup coconut water
- Ice cubes (optional)

Instructions:

1. Combine all ingredients in a blender.

2. Blend until smooth.

3. Pour into a glass, and enjoy!

Nutrition Information:

- Calories: 120
- Protein: 3g
- Carbohydrates: 25g
- Fat: 1g
- Fiber: 5g
- Portion Size: 1 serving

Berry Blast Smoothie

Ingredients:

- 1 cup mixed berries (strawberries, blueberries, raspberries)
- 1 banana
- 1/2 cup Greek yogurt
- 1 tablespoon honey
- 1 cup almond milk
- Ice cubes (optional)

Instructions:

1. Blend all ingredients until creamy.

2. Pour into a glass, and savor the berry goodness.

Nutrition Information:

- Calories: 180
- Protein: 7g
- Carbohydrates: 35g
- Fat: 2g
- Fiber: 6g
- Portion Size: 1 serving

Tropical Paradise Smoothie

Ingredients:

- 1/2 cup pineapple chunks
- 1/2 cup mango chunks
- 1 banana
- 1/2 cup coconut water
- 1/2 cup orange juice
- Ice cubes (optional)

Instructions:

1. Blend all ingredients until smooth.

2. Pour into a glass, and transport yourself to a tropical paradise.

Nutrition Information:

- Calories: 160
- Protein: 2g
- Carbohydrates: 40g
- Fat: 1g
- Fiber: 4g
- Portion Size: 1 serving

Spinach and Pineapple Smoothie

Ingredients:

- 2 cups fresh spinach
- 1 cup pineapple chunks
- 1/2 banana
- 1/2 cup plain Greek yogurt
- 1/2 cup water
- Ice cubes (optional)

Instructions:

1. Blend all ingredients until creamy.

2. Pour into a glass, and relish the green goodness.

Nutrition Information:

- Calories: 140

- Protein: 5g

- Carbohydrates: 30g

- Fat: 1g

- Fiber: 5g

- Portion Size: 1 serving

Cucumber Mint Smoothie

Ingredients:

- 1 cucumber, peeled

- 1/2 cup mint leaves

- 1/2 lime, juiced

- 1 tablespoon agave nectar

- 1 cup coconut water

- Ice cubes (optional)

Instructions:

1. Blend all ingredients until smooth.

2. Pour into a glass, and enjoy the cool, refreshing taste.

Nutrition Information:

- Calories: 90
- Protein: 2g
- Carbohydrates: 20g
- Fat: 1g
- Fiber: 3g
- Portion Size: 1 serving

Chocolate Banana Protein Smoothie

Ingredients:

- 1 banana
- 1 scoop chocolate protein powder
- 1 tablespoon almond butter
- 1 cup milk (dairy or plant-based)
- Ice cubes (optional)

Instructions:

1. Blend all ingredients until well combined.

2. Pour into a glass, and indulge in a protein-packed treat.

Nutrition Information:

- Calories: 250
- Protein: 20g
- Carbohydrates: 25g
- Fat: 10g
- Fiber: 4g
- Portion Size: 1 serving

Mango Coconut Smoothie

Ingredients:

- 1 cup mango chunks
- 1/2 cup shredded coconut
- 1/2 cup Greek yogurt
- 1/2 cup coconut milk
- 1 tablespoon honey
- Ice cubes (optional)

Instructions:

1. Blend all ingredients until smooth and creamy.

2. Pour into a glass, and savor the tropical blend.

Nutrition Information:

- Calories: 220
- Protein: 8g
- Carbohydrates: 30g
- Fat: 9g
- Fiber: 3g
- Portion Size: 1 serving

Blueberry Almond Butter Smoothie

Ingredients:

- 1 cup blueberries
- 2 tablespoons almond butter
- 1/2 banana
- 1 cup almond milk
- 1 tablespoon chia seeds
- Ice cubes (optional)

Instructions:

1. Blend all ingredients until well combined.
2. Pour into a glass, and enjoy the nutty goodness.

Nutrition Information:

- Calories: 230
- Protein: 7g
- Carbohydrates: 28g
- Fat: 11g
- Fiber: 6g
- Portion Size: 1 serving

Kiwi and Kale Smoothie

Ingredients:

- 2 kiwis, peeled and sliced
- 1 cup kale leaves, stems removed
- 1/2 green apple, cored
- 1/2 lime, juiced
- 1 cup water
- Ice cubes (optional)

Instructions:

1. Blend all ingredients until smooth.
2. Pour into a glass, and revel in the vibrant green blend.

Nutrition Information:

- Calories: 120
- Protein: 3g
- Carbohydrates: 30g
- Fat: 1g
- Fiber: 5g
- Portion Size: 1 serving

Orange Creamsicle Smoothie

Ingredients:

- 1 cup orange segments
- 1/2 cup vanilla Greek yogurt
- 1/2 cup orange juice
- 1 tablespoon honey
- 1 cup ice cubes

Instructions:

1. Blend all ingredients until creamy.
2. Pour into a glass, and relish the nostalgic creamsicle flavor.

Nutrition Information:

- Calories: 160
- Protein: 5g
- Carbohydrates: 35g
- Fat: 1g
- Fiber: 3g
- Portion Size: 1 serving

Pomegranate Berry Smoothie

Ingredients:

- 1/2 cup pomegranate seeds
- 1 cup mixed berries (strawberries, blueberries, raspberries)
- 1/2 banana
- 1/2 cup plain Greek yogurt
- 1 cup almond milk
- Ice cubes (optional)

Instructions:

1. Blend all ingredients until smooth.
2. Pour into a glass, and enjoy the antioxidant-rich goodness.

Nutrition Information:

- Calories: 150
- Protein: 6g
- Carbohydrates: 30g
- Fat: 2g
- Fiber: 6g
- Portion Size: 1 serving

Avocado and Spinach Smoothie

Ingredients:

- 1/2 avocado
- 2 cups fresh spinach
- 1/2 cucumber, peeled
- 1/2 lime, juiced
- 1 cup coconut water
- Ice cubes (optional)

Instructions:

1. Blend all ingredients until creamy.
2. Pour into a glass, and revel in the creamy green goodness.

Nutrition Information:

- Calories: 180
- Protein: 5g
- Carbohydrates: 20g
- Fat: 10g
- Fiber: 6g
- Portion Size: 1 serving

Raspberry Chia Seed Smoothie

Ingredients:

- 1 cup raspberries
- 1 tablespoon chia seeds
- 1/2 banana
- 1/2 cup Greek yogurt
- 1 cup almond milk
- Ice cubes (optional)

Instructions:

1. Blend all ingredients until well combined.
2. Pour into a glass, and enjoy the delightful texture of chia seeds.

Nutrition Information:

- Calories: 160
- Protein: 7g
- Carbohydrates: 25g
- Fat: 5g
- Fiber: 8g
- Portion Size: 1 serving

Peanut Butter Banana Smoothie

Ingredients:

- 2 tablespoons peanut butter
- 1 banana
- 1/2 cup oats
- 1 cup milk (dairy or plant-based)
- 1 tablespoon honey
- Ice cubes (optional)

Instructions:

1. Blend all ingredients until smooth.
2. Pour into a glass, and relish the classic combination of peanut butter and banana.

Nutrition Information:

- Calories: 300
- Protein: 12g
- Carbohydrates: 35g
- Fat: 15g
- Fiber: 5g
- Portion Size: 1 serving

Watermelon Mint Smoothie

Ingredients:

- 2 cups diced watermelon
- 1/4 cup fresh mint leaves
- 1/2 lime, juiced
- 1 cup coconut water
- Ice cubes (optional)

Instructions:

1. Blend all ingredients until refreshing and smooth.
2. Pour into a glass, and enjoy the hydrating essence of watermelon.

Nutrition Information:

- Calories: 100
- Protein: 2g
- Carbohydrates: 25g
- Fat: 1g
- Fiber: 3g
- Portion Size: 1 serving

CONCLUSION

In the concluding chapter of this insightful cookbook, we embark on a journey that transcends the realm of recipes. This Chapter is not merely an endpoint but a gateway to understanding, a celebration of newfound culinary wisdom. As we reflect on the flavors explored and the nourishment imparted, it's a moment to savor the victories of embracing a renal-friendly diet.

Within these pages, you'll encounter more than just a summary; this Chapter is a heartfelt narrative, a testament to the transformative power of mindful eating. It whispers encouragement to those who have navigated the delectable landscapes of the previous chapters, urging them to continue this culinary voyage with newfound confidence.

This concluding segment weaves together the threads of experience, emphasizing the broader significance of a renal-conscious lifestyle. It's a space for personal reflections, a pause to acknowledge the growth achieved through each thoughtfully crafted meal. In essence, this Chapter invites you to embrace not just the recipes but the holistic essence of a complete renal diet.

As we bid farewell to this culinary expedition, this Chapter stands as a beacon, illuminating the path towards sustained well-being. It's more than a conclusion; it's a prologue to a continued commitment to health, nourishment, and the joyous art of cooking with purpose.